My Story

My name is Rob (Raw) Maraby

I am a healer, herbalist and the best at what I do (I am not saying this to brag but that is how confident I am in my healing skills).

As a detoxification specialist, I am trained to use fruits & herbs to heal. I am also an avid herbalist and an internet celebrity. I show you how to use fruits and veggies to heal your body. My social media accounts reach over 260,000 people a day and has helped so many people heal them selves naturally.

My principles are very simple; I believe that the cause of man's ills is obstruction of energy flow between the lymph, blood and nerves, this blockage of energy causes poor health. This obstruction is caused by eating the wrong foods not designed for man. And by simply replacing it with the right foods and using herbs, you can greatly boost your well being and health. No supplements are needed, no complicated diet, no vigorous exercise (In fact, this can actually hurt you if you do just one thing incorrectly). All I want from you is to heal.

I discovered natural healing by chance (over 9 years ago), as a bodybuilder with aches and pains. My wife and I went to a raw vegetable retreat for 3 weeks, what I saw and experienced in my health and energy levels changed my life forever. Three years into mostly raw veganism I stumbled onto eating a fruit only diet and eating only fruits, completely healed my body of pains and aches.

I dropped all the excess pounds and water weight that the veggies simply could not take away. I also used fruit to heal my thinning hair and toenail fungus which I had for 20 years (even after treating it with conventional methods). Being so blown away by the results of using fruits and herbs to heal, I decided to share my methods with the world and the response has been overwhelming successfully. This is why I have made it my goal to help others heal.

"You have helped me more in the last several months than my own doctor in the last several years" Raw_ maraby Instagram follower
TESTIMONIALS
These are unsolicited and taken from my social media account comments

How to Heal Yourself Even When They Say You Can't

★ ★ ★ ★ ★

I have been doing this (detox) for a month. A Clean diet...fruits & vegetables...and the effect is excellent. I don't have much appetite -my hunger is less and my energy is high...better skin too

-@deepbainsdb

★ ★ ★ ★ ★

"Thanks to you I've been getting in shape and eating healthier...dude my hair is growing like crazy and my skin and nails look healthy..."

-@dominican_dragon

★ ★ ★ ★ ★

"I started all fruits 4 days ago. I'm surprised by how good I feel already. I am not hungry or craving anything, not bloated, my post nasal drip and sinus issues have stopped..."

- Kathy Mattheu

How to Heal Yourself Even When They Say You Can't

By Mourab (Raw) Maraby- Certified detox specialist and herbalist.

Before We Start: Here Is A Medical Disclaimer.

As you will soon find out I don't believe in diseases so this book is not about diseases but about natural healing. Diseases to me are symptoms of a deep underlying cause and so we always address the deep cause and never the disease. So this book is not about treating or curing, but about healing and getting well. Always see your doctor to treat or cure a disease.

So all content found in this book including: text, images, audio, or other formats were created for informational purposes only. The content is not intended to be a substitute for professional medical advice, diagnosis, or treatment.

If you think you may have a medical emergency, call your doctor, go to the emergency department, or call 911 immediately. The author does not recommend or endorse any specific tests, physicians, products, procedures, opinions, or other information that may be mentioned on here. Reliance on any information provided here is solely at your own risk.

The Content in this book is provided on an "as is" basis. Use at your own risk

Why I wrote this book

How to become healthy again when everything you have tried in the past has failed you. I wrote this book to show you a simple way to go from 'hell-ville' (a state of unhealthy or ill health to a state of 'well-ville' (good health) using nothing but fruits and plants. II know it sounds crazy, as we are coming from a world of science but the truth is when it comes to good health Mother Nature is still the best. Nothing works when it is complicated and nature is simple. It is very complex at the deeper level but its function is simple.

I can say this if you follow my steps and put everything you think about health aside you are going to be very surprised and pleased at the results. All you need to do is give it 2-

3 weeks and I am certain that you would get a wonderful result and people will equally see it and benefit from your experience.

I knew I had to get this in the hands of every man, woman, and child.

And I wrote this in a way that even a child can read it, understand it and use it to help anyone. I did not write this to show you theories and why I think something works. I know from helping thousands that this really works and that you only have to try it and see.

Let's be honest, everywhere you look there is another fad diet or another doctor selling you a probiotic or detox drink. All this is a bit too much, I know for me and my clients, we really just want something that really works to get us better and here it is. I poured my heart into this and wrote without holding back. So read, educate yourself and then take control of your health and all that comes with it.

Grandma and mother always said "eat your fruits and veggies"
They also used to say "an apple a day keeps the doctor away"
This has been passed from one generation to another and there is a golden key to health in it and I am about to give you this key.

It is the key to health, vitality, happiness, and spirituality and it is here in this book. if you put aside all doubts and try it, I am telling you it is going to be the best gift you ever got and this book is going to be PRICELESS and you will want to give a copy to everyone you care about.

I wrote this book to help you heal. My goal in this book is not to use scientific jargon, nor is it to show off with scientific studies.

Because sometimes studies can be skewed to show results to whoever is paying for those results.

I don't believe in diseases, I believe that <u>every disease is a symptom of obstruction</u> of one or many of the main energy flows of the body- lymph flow, blood flow, and nerve flow. And when you address the cause of these obstructions you allow the body to heal itself and allow yourself to live a youthful and healthy life- just as nature intended you to... I believe healing is simple, so simple even a child could do it.

We are living breathing beings made of energy and knowing this we can all get well if we eat foods that resonate and provide this energy (raw fruits and veggies).

My ideas here are real and the proof is in you- I mean when you use these tips you will see the proof, in fact, there are very few people this would not work for.

And it would not work because these people will not go through with the principles or give it some time to work.

If you have a health issue that has been with you for a decade or more surely you need to give the body some time to heal. You can't expect healing to show up overnight when the condition is chronic or degenerative. Remember there are miles and miles of lymph fluids, capillaries, and blood vessels all through the body and it takes time to get them to run efficiently and effectively.

Everyone has some theory and as humans, we want a quick fix and so we buy the next fad or the next theory by some wonderful scientists but you and I both know they don't work.

So what I will share with you is practical and you need only prove it to yourself.

First of all, the cause of your issues is the obstruction of energy flow. In the body you have energy flowing via blood, via nerves and via lymph and when any one of these are blocked the body will become inflamed- this inflammation becomes symptoms and pains and because we don't understand what's going on we run to the doctor to get medicine to take the pain away, this medicine just suppresses and hides the main cause and this leads to a serious problem later on.

I am all for medical doctors but this book is not about treating or curing - it is about healing the root cause of the health issue.

You really can't treat a health issue and hope it won't come back again. Treatment is just what it is- a treatment- it is not a fix. It is a band-aid policy.

So in natural healing, we go after the cause of the issue and by so doing **we allow the body to heal itself** which it does perfectly well.

My philosophy, in a nutshell, is this: The cause of man's health issues is due to obstructions of energy flow *(lymph flow, nerve flow, and blood flow) and one becomes healthy by removing these obstructions:*

Obstructions are caused by:
Not eating foods designed for man (cooked foods, starches and animal products)
Poor food combining (you can't mix proteins and starches if you want good digestion)
Too much food (the human body needs little food when clean and unobstructed)

Toxins (pollution will affect the body and energy pathways).
A disruption in the mucus membrane – the mucus membrane is a lining that protects and covers the surface of internal organs, when it is compromised or broken by acids and or obstruction a health issue is created and a symptom is shown by the body in that specific location

How to Heal Yourself Even When They Say You Can't

A symptom is an indication from the body that there is obstruction of energy flow

In my opinion whatever health issue you have, it's caused by obstruction. e.g. Tumors are obstruction of lymph. And nerve issues are the obstruction of lymph and nerve flow.

So common sense tells you that to get healthy you need to first clean the cells and then re-energize the cells and we do this with fruits and herbs- I know it sounds too simple to work but I can tell you that if you just try it you will see for yourself how simple it is to get healthy

Remember that healing is simple and never complicated.

There are 4 stages of disease and 4 stages of wellness as well.

Before I discuss the 4 stages of dis-eases and the 4 stages of wellness let me get a few points across to help you understand.

Humans are frugivorous- meaning we eat fruits. We are closest in relationship to the ape – they eat fruits in their natural environment, when pushed into an unnatural environment they will eat insects and greens otherwise they are frugivorous, we too are frugivorous, there is nothing in us that is aggressive, we don't look
at an animal and say "yummy" let me eat it or tear it apart. But we will look at ripe fruits and salivate.

Someone people say well we have 2 carnivore teeth...these are teeth meant to be use to bite and tear at fruits and nothing else. Like a can opener.

We don't have fangs like a carnivore does and when we eat foods that are alien to our bodies like processed foods, cooked foods, animal products we create an immune or mucosa response and they body begins to find ways of dealing with these alien foods, the end results is hardening of mucus and plaguing from...

When we eat foods we were designed for -fruits and veggies there is no obstructions

Step 2
Your body is pretty made up of a bunch of cells and two fluids. I don't care what part of the body you test or take from, it is a bunch of cells; even bones are a bunch of cells. Now while all these cells have different and complex functions they all do two things

1. They consume nutrients and
2. They eliminate waste (acids or metabolic waste) from those nutrients

Now to feed the cells, the blood comes in and does that job and to remove waste the body uses the lymphatic system which is the main sewer system or immune system of the body.

The blood makes about 25% of the fluids in a cell and the lymph makes about 75% off the fluids in a cell. (This does not factor in water content)

And this makes sense because we all have the capacity to eliminate waste should be greater than the capacity to consume foods- if not there will be a blockage or overflow.

Medical science does not recognize the function of the lymphatic system and so this is where the difficulty in treating diseases comes because they don't know what the real cause of these so called dis-eases are. - It is the great lymphatic system

So what exactly is lymph?

Lymph is a cholesterol or lipid based fatty liquid. Its job is to protect the cells from acid waste, it is also its job to remove waste and pass it through the lymph nodes where it is then passed through to the kidneys and then the bladder to be eliminated as urine.

 The lymph system does not have a pump like the blood and so it requires activity to move. Gentle exercises like walking, running and yoga do a great job of moving lymph. Lymph moves well when we are eating the right alkaline foods (fruits and vegetables) but they move poorly when we eat starches, animal products and cooked foods.

Lymph waste from cells will always pass through a lymph node.

lymph nodes are the body's septic tank when your cells excrete waste these wastes are acidic in nature and these acids have to be neutralized by something otherwise the acids could burn the kidneys and other important organs and glands.

The body uses the lymph nodes which are like "septic tanks" to neutralize these acids.

Why did we compare it to a septic tank? Well, it is because in all septic tanks there will always be bacteria in it. Bacteria is good because it "eats" acids and wastes and converts them into lesser acids.

So similarly, in these lymph nodes, there are bacteria whose job it is to eat those acids and convert it into a lesser aggressive acid. Its job is to break down sewage waste.

Once treated into lesser acids, the lymphatic system takes these less acidic wastes to the kidneys to be eliminated - the kidneys are therefore the sewage plant of the body. Their jobs are to remove those acids from the lymph system and expel it to the outside world.

Your kidneys may not be working well.

Why? The foods we eat – the cooked starches and the animal products will harden and burden the lymphatic system and the kidneys, the work becomes too much that they don't work as well.

Now, what happens when the kidneys are not filtering properly?

Think about your house, when you flush the toilet and the toilet is clogged what happens?

Answer: It backs up and overflows

When your kidneys are not filtering properly as they should, acids will back up and these will cause cells and the fluids in them to get hard and dry, lymph nodes will swell, fluids (blood, lymph, and nerve flow) won't flow properly and nutrients will not be easily delivered to cells.
Also, cells won't be able to communicate with the brain or CNS (central nervous system) or PNS (peripheral nervous system) the result is cellular damage and degeneration. With regards to nerves, you can get a host of nervous system health issues. This includes loss of memories, breathing problems, dizziness, and lack of automatic movements.

The body will become stiff, hard and there will be inflammation, pain, and swelling. Organs and glands will stop working properly and you will wonder what is going on (does all this sound familiar?). And if ignored cells will eventually begin to get destroyed and degenerate if you do not get rid of those acids.

How to tell if your kidneys are not filtering

If you wake up in the morning pee into a clear jar, you should see some sediment in the urine, it should have strings in it or cloudy like particles. If you see this you are filtering. If not you are not filtering effectively. This fruit detox program will help get your kidneys filtering.

If your urine is not clear and has strands or sediment in it, it means the body is removing metabolic waste from the cells. (That is good). The more sediment you see the better if you see the urine is clear this means your kidneys are not filtering properly and you are likely to have acids come through your skin in the form of rashes, redness and other skin issues.

If your kidneys are not filtering you need to go on a 100% fruits only diet. It has to be nothing but 100% raw fruits.

Stop eating cooked and processed foods and stop eating any animal products as these are highly acidic and will damage the lymphatic system and kidneys.
Replace these foods with hydrating and alkalizing fruits and veggies.
Use herbs that help the kidneys and lymphatic system work better – for kidneys, the best are parsley, dandelion and corn silk.

For the lymphatic system chaparral is the best.

Use some dry fasting (no food and no water) to help give the body a chance to repair and clean itself.

You should know that often the kidneys will respond right away but more often than not they won't and you should not give up, just stay on fruits and veggies and they will filter eventually. I will discuss this later and show you how to get your kidneys working and filtering.
Remember this is not a race; it is not about who finishes first but who finishes. Health is a journey and not a competition.

Acids versus bases and your health

In nature and in life, all chemistry is divided into an acid or base. There are two sides of chemistry; there is an acid and a base side to chemistry.

It does not matter what element you look at it is either an acid or a base.

Now acids are burning, dehydrating, drying, hot, destroyers, they harden things and destroy. Let's think of it as the male or aggressive side of chemistry.

The base is the cooling, hydrating, pleasant, healthy, free-flowing side of chemistry let's call it the female side of chemistry.

The body is predominantly alkaline or base in composition.

And when we consume foods and it is digested the food either leaves acid ash or an alkaline ash deposit. This means the foods we eat will either help the body stay alkaline or turn it acidic.

Acids and bases are opposite of each other. They neutralize one another. It is a bit like pouring vinegar into baking soda, you will see that there is a reaction as the acid (vinegar) is neutralized by the base (baking soda)

The same thing happens to the body at all levels.

The human body is predominantly alkaline and has to be kept that way. When we consume acid ash foods, this balance is affected and imbalance is created and the body has to fight hard to neutralize these acids and maintain an alkaline balance. So when we eat acid ash foods the following happens:

Cholesterol is produced by the body to fight these acids (creates plaque or obstruction) The body takes calcium from cell walls and tissue to fight these acids- this creates weak veins and bones.

The lymphatic system backs up and gets hard and clogged like a stagnated river.

The acids are hard on the kidneys which affect the lymphatic system as well.

The body becomes hard, cells get damaged and nutrients don't get to cells effectively and the result is health issues, symptoms of pain and inflammation begin to accumulate.

It seems simple, doesn't it? We simply have to eat foods that allow the body to be alkaline and stop eating foods that make the body acidic.
When the body becomes too acidic we call it ACIDOSIS and this leads to inflammation (immune response) and then health issues. This is the underlying cause of health issues.

It does not matter what it is, this is the primary and overlooked cause.
Symptoms are the body's way of telling you that the body is acidic and is failing (in flames), you can treat it and hope it will go away; you need to remove and address the underlying cause of ill health.

You don't have a cholesterol problem, you have an acid problem.
And cholesterol does not coat the inside of an artery, it coats in between the cell walls and in between cells which leads to a swelling of the artery and a clogging of blood flow. So as you can see, treating it does not do much as it does not address the cause - **ACIDOSIS**.

Dis-eases and health issues

What are they? People call it disease and treat it like it is something that we catch when in effect it is simply a cause and effect. Garbage in, garbage out. What we eat is what manifests in our body-it is that simple.

What we eat, drink, breathe and smell has an effect on the body, if it's acidic or acid ash it will affect the PH balance of the body and create health issues.

Well is it my mum and dad's fault?

When we eat foods that are alien to the body, the body has an immediate immune response or mucosa response. What is mucus?

Mucus covers and protects every cell and tissue. It is a slippery fatty substance to protect cells from outside factors, so when we eat foods alien to the body, a mucosa response is triggered and you get a runny nose or, pain, fever or coughing.

Most people when they experience these immediate reactions will take medication to suppress these responses and the result is that the body will push these wastes and alien foods into the body (cells) and it will create an obstruction and worsen things.

What is suppressed is tomorrow's nightmare

In reality, when you have such a response, you want to make all attempts to expel and help the body eliminate these mucus and obstructive foods.

Think about your house. If you don't throw out the garbage and keep piling it up, your house is going to smell, insects and animals will get into the house and eventually the entire house will rot. The body is the same way

So a general rule is if you get an immune response, don't stop the cold or flu response, but rather help the body get it out and stop consuming the foods that are causing these responses.

Antibiotics?

The usual cause of action from your doctor when you get a cold is to give you antibiotics and while this can be good when you are desperately in need of some sort of relief. But these antibiotics might harm helpful bacteria. Bacteria is nature's soldiers, their job is to break down waste, their job is to clean, you have bacteria in your gut which gets affected by antibiotics, you have bacteria in your lymph nodes without which you will have a hard time eliminating acids from the cells.

We have bacteria all over and in our bodies, it is natural and actually healthy if you are eating the right foods and have a strong lymphatic system and kidneys. And this book is designed to get all the organs and cells of your body healthy so they can maintain and invite the right bacteria needed for healthy living.

Don't add probiotics or added bacteria to your gut if you are not filtering through your kidneys or if you are not well. Adding these bacteria is not wise as it adds to the bacteria load and the body can't handle it.

And here is the crucial piece of the pie, if you actually kill bacteria who is going to break down your waste?

Put it another way, if your septic tank has no bacteria it won't work properly.

4 stages of diseases

Dis-ease or health issues don't just happen. It takes a while to get to a chronic condition. For instance, if you have arthritis it did not just happen. It went through a series of steps and these steps were ignored until it hit the chronic stage and in which case the pain was too much to ignore.

So let's discuss the 4 stages of sickness. These are just broad stages, each stage has further sub-stages but we don't need to know this as you can heal without it and healing is the goal and not complex thinking or intellectualism.

As I mentioned earlier we are frugivorous (Fruit eaters) and the foods we are designed to eat are fruits. These foods are the natural human food and when we eat foods, not in the fruit category and veggies category we put an acid hit on the body. This means the body becomes acidic when we eat foods that are not designed for humans. The response to this is that the body uses mucus to protect itself from this acid hit the body is predominantly alkaline and when we eat acid causing foods the causes acidosis - and things in the body go from being alkaline, hydrated and supple to dry, hardened and a cationic environment - which causes diseases.

Stage 1
Acute stage- you usually get a runny nose, phlegm build up, coughing and cold and flu-like symptoms.

Stage 2
This is the sub-acute stage of disease

We usually don't see anything wrong with a little runny nose or a cold or flu-like symptom so we ignore it or suppress it with medication and we continue eating the foods that caused the problem in the first place. And as we consume these foods and continue to ignore this mucosa response by suppressing it with medication or by eating more of the acid foods (ignoring cause and effect) the mucus buries itself deeper and deeper in the cells of the body and it begins to harden and become obstructive to energy flow (blood flow, lymph flow, and nerve flow)

Stage 3

Chronic stage
the third stage is the chronic stage and at this stage the mucus is imposing on cells and it creates a hyper or hypo activity in glands and organs, in chronic stages the glands and organs switch from hyper to hypofunction and everything is going down, this leads to chronic dis-eases like arthritis, fibromyalgia, lupus, and loss of calcium these

symptoms are the effects of chronic acidosis. Your body has become too acidic and when nothing is done further it leads to stage 4.

Stage 4

Degenerative stage
The final stage is the degenerative state –this state is often called the cancer states and at this stage, the acids are burning the cells from within- intracellular acidosis – It causes mutation

Signs of the stages
Acute- and subacute stages

Cold and flu-like symptoms, fever, sweating, coughing up mucus, vomiting, diarrhea. Mucus you spit out is white to yellow

Chronic and degenerative states, - mucus is green and brown (chronic health issues)

Degenerative states- mucus is black (degenerative pain and dis-eases)

If you are not detoxing you will not see the chronic and degenerative signs, because they are only visible when you detox and the deeper you go into the body the more you are likely to see the signs of ill health come out of the body. The acute and sub-acute stages you tend to see visible signs when you eat mucus causing foods like dairy products or animal products you tend to spit out white mucus or when you have a runny nose in the initial stages of eating these foods.

Also, when you detox they start healing backward, you will start regenerating that which is degenerating first . You will go from the chronic stages then move to the subacute stages and then the acute level. In this process, you can relive every injury you had in the past

Detoxification

Detoxification is simply cleaning all the mess that you put in your body or that the body put in there in an attempt to (hardened mucus to protect itself from acids) protect itself.

It is simple to fix what we have made unhealthy:
The acute and subacute stages are easy to fix and take less time to fix the chronic and

degenerative stages are harder but you will see remarkable progress in a few weeks on 100% fruits and herbs. However, remember that if you ignore the acute and subacute phases, (when you continue eating more acid ash causing food like starches and animal products) the kidneys will stop filtering and cause a block of energy flow. And that leads to burying and hardening of mucus in between cells and this starts the further descent into the chronic and degenerative states. This is a very simple cause and effect situation.

Again, you can heal the body. All you do is simply stop eating the foods causing the acidosis and replace with 100% raw fruits and veggies and you will feel the difference almost instantly- usually in a day or two. This is the proof you need and no one regrets going into a fruit and veggie diet.

The proof lies in you- I am saying you be the proof. You apply the knowledge here and see what happens to your health. It never fails.

The 4 stages of wellness.

To make sure you are healthy, you need to understand these simple 4 stages of wellness. If any of these stages are not functioning properly or are obstructed by a disruption of energy flow or the breakdown of the mucosa membrane there will be health issues. I like to call it obstruction of energy flow. There are three major energy flows, lymph flow, blood flow, and nerve flow and if any of these are blocked there will be inflammation, and pain and acidosis. Don't worry it is not complicated and you don't need to know how it all works, you just need to know the stages and how to use herbs to help you fix the organs and glands in these stages.

The 4 steps to wellness will ensure there are no obstructions to health.

Digestion: You must digest what you put into your mouth. When you put food in your mouth the pancreas will produce enzymes to digest this food.

The liver and gallbladder will also aid in metabolizing fats, proteins, and carbohydrates. You need to break down the foods you put into your mouth before you can absorb it through the stomach and small intestines.

The pancreas and the liver are the gland and the organ responsible for digesting food. If they are not well or functioning properly you will not be able to digest food properly and you will see undigested food in your stool.

The liver is like a giant factory that produces all the functional needs of the body. Its basic and essential tasks are amino acid metabolism, carbohydrate metabolism as well as fat metabolism. So we have to make sure that the digestive glands and organs are working properly and we do this by going on a fruit diet and using herbs for the pancreas (endocrine system) and the liver and gall bladder. If the food you eat does not properly digest, you will become unhealthy.

Absorption: Once the food is digested into nutrients, these nutrients have to be absorbed by the small intestine. If your intestines are clogged by mucoid plaque or congested (interstitial lymphatic constipation) you will not be able to absorb nutrients.

Interstitial lymphatic constipation will cause mal-absorption. The GI tract is the system responsible for absorption. It is the hub of your body and when it is not working properly it causes constipation and mal-absorption; this can weaken and actually starve your body.

The issues you may get when your GI tract is inflamed or not functioning properly is that it sets up a terrain for parasites, bacteria, and worms. There is mal-absorption and constipation. And worse still when clogged toxins leach back into the blood and cause health issues and blood poisoning. Lymphatic congestion leads to improper cellular elimination. And what you don't eliminate you will accumulate.

Utilization: Once the nutrients have been absorbed they have to be utilized and the gland that does this is the adrenal glands. They are two of them on top of each kidney and their job is to produce corticosteroids that allow minerals to be used in the body they also produce hormones that ensure proper nerve communication between cells and is in control of fight or flight mechanisms and automatic movements like breathing and using the washroom.

The adrenal's produce neurotransmitters which are essential for proper brain and nerve function- e.g. it produces neurotransmitters like epinephrine and adrenaline as well as **Norepinephrine** and dopamine, which affect the sympathetic and parasympathetic nervous system – which are the two autonomic nervous systems of the body. Remember that the nerves of the body control movement and many other communications between cells as well, so you want this to be healthy.

Elimination:

The next step is elimination. Are you eliminating properly? This includes digestive waste (stool) and lymphatic waste (metabolic waste). If you don't eliminate waste, your body becomes congested and acidic, the acids begin to affect cells (tissue, organs, and glands) and the dis-ease processes that we are familiar with comes into effect.

The kidneys and the skin are the key organs responsible for removing metabolic waste, and the bowels are responsible for getting rid of digestive waste.

The most overlooked cause of health issues is lymphatic congestion, meaning you can't eliminate waste through your lymphatic system and through to your kidneys.

The Key To Health Is A Healthy Lymphatic System

This is the main sewer system of the body, picture a sewer system all through an entire city and if this system breaks the whole city is going to get damaged because the waste from its citizens have nowhere to go and it will rot homes, start degradation and allow parasites to breed and thrive.

The lymphatic system removes the wastes from your 100 trillion cells and if they are not moving properly these acids from your 100 trillion cells back up and begin to burn cells.

And when the lymphatic system is not working properly the kidneys stop working as well and this means the wastes have nowhere to go and often try to make it through the skin (the third kidney).

The kidneys are the sewage plant of the body, its job is to process the acids brought by the lymphatic system and then store it in the bladder then eliminated through urine. Again this part is crucial to understanding why you get health issues.

For instance if you have a weak or damaged thyroid, you can't really fix the thyroid unless you fix the lymphatic system and the kidneys, because the damage caused to the thyroid is done by acids which can't be removed by the lymphatic system and the kidneys. If you treat the thyroid it is only a temporary solution but does not address the cause which are acids burning the thyroid or some other gland that controls the thyroid like the pituitary gland.

So how does one get healthy?

If you have issues of any of the 4 processes to wellness above, how do you fix it?

Well here are the golden steps:

1. Change your diet to an alkaline diet- raw fruits and veggies are like firemen, they will put out fires in the body. The fires in the body are acids causing inflammation (burning) and the firemen hydrate the body and alkalize the body. Next stop eating the foods causing the fires, a: these are cooked foods and animal products. In fact, it includes everything except raw fruits and vegetables.

2. Detox the acids and hardened mucus out. Use dry fasting and raw fruits, raw veggies and fresh or dried herbs to clean out the obstructions and acids in the body

3. Rebuild tissue with herbs, raw fruits, and raw veggies.

How to Heal Yourself Even When They Say You Can't

Herbs

Herbs- Hippocrates the father of medicine said: **"let food be your medicine and medicine be your food"** that is a very simple and powerful teaching. Note that food does not include synthetic and manmade products and foods; it is literally raw fruit and veggies. **Here is a secret to health, eat nothing but raw fruits and veggies to heal.** It is kind of like an apple a day keeps the doctor away. It is a half-truth because people take it to mean you can eat anything you want to provided you eat an apple a day you will be healthy.

No...it means eat nothing but fruits and veggies and you will heal. This looks simple right? **It is so simple a child can use this to heal anyone or anything.**

Herbs are a gift from nature, just like fruits or veggies. They have been in existence since the earth was able to grow plants. There are herbs for just about every part of the human body, it is actually quite fascinating

Herbs are all natural and contain natural chemicals and nutrients that help human tissue heal. They strengthen and energize tissue. They are like medicine for the cells. Herbs strengthen the cells. Herbs have energy that is transmitted to the cells and revives them. They affect tissue in a unique way, the plants have synergistic components in them that affect cells, and science does not know the actual reason how and why they work but we do know they work really well with no side effects

In short, herbs are there to help our tissues clean, strengthen and rebuild the health of tissues.

With my healing, we Clean, Strengthen and Rebuild, using fruits, veggies, herbs, and dry fasting. Simple isn't it?

What foods should we eat?

Every animal eats food raw. There is not a single animal in existence that does not eat raw food. Every animal eats foods that are designed for it. Carnivores eat raw meat, humans are the only animals that think we are smarter than nature and tend to eat foods alien to our body.

As humans we are frugivores. We are designed to eat fruits the animal closest to us are primates and they are frugivorous, they eat fruits. So when we eat food alien to us, we begin to get sick. When we eat cooked foods and dress them up with chemicals we get ill, because these are not foods designed for the human body and the body has to make an attempt to fix it and eliminate it

Some people argue that we have a pair of canine teeth so we should eat meat but that is simply untrue, there is nothing in us that allows us to hunt and eat and animal uncooked. So people say we are civilized animals and have more intelligence and hence can cook food but all these acids created from cooked foods only make us ill.

Are we smarter than nature? The answer is no.
And yet we keep eating and drinking cooked, processed and animal products as food and we are getting sicker, fatter, depressed and dis-eases have become more rampant than before the rise of mass consumption of cooked and processed foods.

If you study the human body you will see that we are frugivorous. We don't have lots of long canine teeth, in fact, our pair of canine teeth is only there to rip into fruits much like a can opener, and it is not long enough to pierce into raw flesh. Secondly, our digestive system is only 12 times the length of our spine and we chew with an up and down motion. Hence we are frugivores.

Now I am not here to prove that we are frugivorous, I am here to show you how to heal. So just give me the benefit of the doubt because the proof is in the theory- meaning that if you apply what I teach here you will see healing take place and you will believe and understand why you are a frugivore.

You can take the table test
If you put a plate of ripe fruits on a table, a plate of raw meat, a plate of grass and a plate of nuts and a plate of vegetables and invite a bunch of kids not mentally brainwashed by society, the kids will instinctively go for the fruits. They will never go for the meat. And get this, if we were truly meat eaters, if we saw an animal we would drool but we don't do that. If we see fresh ripe fruits we will always drool because it is delicious and we are instinctively drawn to it

Food is energy for the body
When you eat food, you are transferring energy from one plane to another. The scientist knows that energy is neither created nor destroyed, it is simply transferred.

Energy can be measured in electromagnetic waves called Angstroms. The more angstrom a food has, the higher its energy.

When the body is in good health, it has an angstrom measurement of 6500 angstroms. A person who is sick or has cancer has an angstrom level of 4875 angstroms

So when you eat raw fruits and veggies the high electromagnetic food is transferred and used by your body. This simply means, if you eat life you get life.

Just to get an idea of the angstroms you get from the different foods you eat, let me show you a few examples
Raw fruits (8000-10000 **Angstroms**)
Raw veggies (8000-9000 angstroms)

Honey, raw milk and eggs (3000-5000 **Angstroms**)
Weak angstrom- cooked milk, jams, cheeses (1800), white four (1000 angstroms) and cooked veggies (1500 **Angstroms**)

There is virtually no angstroms is cooked meat (0 **Angstroms**) so it creates negative energy to the body as the body uses more energy than it gets when digesting and eliminating meat and other low energy foods include alcohol, margarine, and refined sugars

So, if you knew you could charge the body and its cells, would you use a low or high angstrom food?

The answer is obvious "No!" – And that is one reason why we use raw fruits to heal. We are pushing energy into the cells to allow it to heal and at the same time we are giving it the least obstructive food to use to heal (remember that it takes energy to digest food).

In short, you create health issues in your body and the good news is that if you caused it, you can change it.
So stop eating the foods causing an obstruction and eat food designed for humans (fruits and veggies).
Watch what you breathe
Watch what you drink

Why eat fruits?

Fruits contain fructose which is a simple sugar that feeds every cell in the body and it is very easy to digest
Fruits possess all the amino acids your body needs to build muscle.
Fruits carry fiber which is great for brushing the colon and bowel walls
Fruits have essential fatty acids
Fruits help cells to regenerate tissue
Fruits are very hydrating to cells and alkalize the body
Fruits feed neurons and they revitalize the brain cells and nerves as well

Fruit is an astringent
It has no mucus that can seal the colon and intestinal walls.
It powers neurons
It's so simple the body won't work hard to digest
 -Its sugar enters cells by diffusion (not with insulin)
- It has flavonoids
- Antioxidants
- It has no karma or violence to eating it (fruits fall off of tree when ripe)
- It's peaceful and anyone who eats it becomes calm and loving.
- It's great for prayer or meditation as it is light
 -it's the purest form of carbon and oxygen (fuel for cells)

- It's sweet
- Everyone who can eat it loves it
It has no mucus or negative mucosa response.

Fruits and diabetes:

People have a bad understanding of diabetes and fruits. But fruits contain fructose and fructose does not need insulin to enter the cells, they enter the cells by diffusion. Meats, cooked starches require insulin and are what causes diabetes and not fruit.

Fruits and cancer

Some people say that sugars feed cancer and that the sugar in fruits feed cancer. This is nonsense – all cells need carbon and sugar is a source of carbon and oxygen and without sugar, the cell dies. A cancer cell is an abnormal or dying cell. You can't take away sugar from cells healthy or unhealthy as this will lead to cell death. So you can't starve a body of sugar -it is impossible. Vegetables, proteins and starches all have sugar and so the statement that sugar feeds cancer is absurd. You need sugar (carbon and oxygen) to feed and sustain cells.

And fruits are the only thing that can remove the lymphatic obstructions that prevent the body from removing abnormal cells.

So what causes diabetes as far as natural healing is concerned?

Obstructions of energy flow within and to the pancreas and adrenals.

The adrenals are responsible for producing neurotransmitters and cortical steroids which allow proper communication between cells tissue and glands, the adrenals also handle sugar metabolism. When you can't metabolize sugar properly, your sugar levels will go up or down. Scientists have found that often insulin is not produced by the pancreas, not because of the pancreas inability to produce insulin but because the nerves in the pancreas are obstructed and can't get messages from the adrenals and pituitary gland (obstruction of nerve flow) and this is why in natural healing we work on the adrenals as well as the pancreas to make sure that it is sending the right signals to the pancreas to produce insulin.

Also note that the adrenals sit on the kidneys and so when adrenals are weak kidneys are weak and when kidneys are weak, the lymphatic system becomes weak as well. You can see that everything is interconnected.

To heal stop eating cooked starches and proteins
You need to consume fruits and herbs and nothing else if you want to detoxify and cleanse the body towards good health.

A few pointers about diabetes and natural healing:

The key energy driver of a cell is carbon and oxygen, every cell needs this to function. Because when you can give a cell carbon and oxygen, ATP is formed and that's energy and vitality for the cell. Cell death occurs when there is no energy being supplied and so as a diabetic, it's crucial you get carbon into your cells. Glucose and other sugars need insulin to supply this carbon to the cell and if you are not producing insulin this poses a problem. **That is why fruits are essential to a diabetic because the carbon is transferred to the cell by diffusion and not insulin.**

If you go on fruits initially you are likely to sugar load for a few days this is not due to the fruits, it is due to the body adjusting to the clean source of energy. Remember that fruit sugars enter the cell by diffusion and need little or no insulin. Complex starches and sugars from proteins need insulin to make their way into a call. This is why you will sugar load with starches and proteins. Even vegetables need insulin. Fruit sugars do not.

So once you get on 100% fruits you are likely to sugar load for 3-4 days- so simply monitor your sugar 10-12 times a day.

Eat small frequent meals of fruit-eating every two hours is a good way to do it
Consume berries as they are very good for detoxing- the glands responsible for poor insulin production (the pancreas).

After 3-4 days on 100% fruits, you will see a drop in blood sugar and then stabilization. You have to see your doctor and adjust your medication accordingly. And eventually you can wean off medication as you and your doctor sees fit.

Avoid fats when detoxing with Diabetes as they create insulin resistance.
Avoid oils and refined sugars (This does not include fruit sugars).
Avoid processed foods like flour and rice.
Unprocessed cooked foods such as baked sweet potatoes, cooked vegetables and quinoa are ok in moderation. Ideally when healing you use 100% raw fruits and nothing else.
There is a tincture or herbs you can use called Glucose formula (See the resource section below)

Here are the herbs used in the Glucose formula. You can make a tea from them here:

Goldenseal Root
Bitter Melon
Devil's Club Root
Fenugreek Seed
Gentian Root
Gymnema Leaf
Hawthorn Berry
Kelp Frond Powder
Myrrh
Parsley Leaf
Pau d'Arco Bark
Prickly Ash Bark
Suma Root
Wild Yam Root

Remember you can't heal your pancreas and adrenals (gland responsible for sugar metabolism with dead foods like cooked starches and animal products) you need high energy raw living foods and herbs.

Here is why you won't want to consume meat

Meats are complex protein structures and they are extremely hard to digest. They are full of stimulants, steroids, and antibiotics that affect your glands and organs. The protein in meat is not designed for human consumption. When meat is digested it leaves an acid ash deposit and the body takes an acid hit and this affects the alkalinity of the body.

The proteins from meat are very irritating to the mucosa of the body. It elicits an immune response that the body uses mucus to protect itself from the consumption of meat.

Meat can create body odor when consumed.

Meat eaters are very aggressive due to the karmic nature of meat together with the stimulants and steroids in the meat

Eating meat has been shown to be a big factor in diabetes and intestinal and colon cancer.

Meat is very hard on the kidneys and will affect the lymphatic system.

You can get all the amino acids from fruits and veggies and you don't want meat protein.
If there is one thing you should avoid, it is meat. It is like slow poison and anyone who recommends high protein or lots of meat is clueless about healing the body.

How About Dairy Products

Humans are not designed to drink milk, even mothers milk is hard to digest, However because we produce enzymes to digest mothers milk we can use mother milk for a few years. However, after the age of 2 these enzymes are not produced anymore, so when we drink milk after the age of 2 it creates a mucus response and causes lymphatic congestion. You can feel the effects of eating them by its mucosa response.

When we continue to consume dairy whiles ignoring the mucosa response the body suppresses the mucosa response and stores the hardened dairy it can't digest on the bowel walls and a mucoid plaque is created. This prevents proper absorption and can create autoimmune health issues as these undigested toxic food seeps into the bloodstream.

The congestion created by dairy products will affect the thyroid and parathyroid and affect the production of hormones, these glands will eventually begin to fail and it is a vicious cycle of ill health and weakening of tissue, organs, and glands.

Drinking milk creates acidity in the body which will cause the body to leech of calcium from cell walls and use that to neutralize acids. It is ironic to think that milk is promoted as a source of calcium when it actually steals calcium from the body.

How about grains and beans? They are good right?

No, they are not. Grains and beans are sleeping foods; they contain special enzymes around them that prevent the seeds from germinating. Only when they are washed in water do they get activated and then have to sprout before they are edible and become a vegetable. But beans and grains are not edible food.. They are hard to digest and rob the body of energy – this means more energy is used to digest it than it gives the body.

Beans and grains are acid forming foods, this means once consumed they leave an acid as a deposit which affects the acidity level of the body and will affect the lymphatic system and the kidneys.

Soybeans are not also good, they are marketed as a good source of healthy nutrients but it is far from the truth. Soy milk is estrogenic, it is high in enzyme inhibitors and the majority of the soy on the market is genetically modified foods (GMO).
The way soy milk is extracted makes it toxic and possibly cancerous.

How about fats?
Animal fats, vegetable oils like soy canola, corn are all acidic. They are hard to digest and very complex in nature and structure, this means the body has to break it down and it leaves acid ash by-product, they affect the kidneys and lymphatic system

We do need good fats and you can get them from raw fruits and veggies.
Good fats will help insulate cells.
They will be stored and used as a source of energy.
They assist with the creation of steroids and hormones used for utilizing vitamins and minerals.
Fats are anti-inflammatory and protect the cells and neutralize acids in the body.
Fats make up the majority of the lymphatic system.

How about sugars?
Sugar is the main source of carbon for your body. We are carbon beings and we need energy in the form of sugar. Simple sugars are the primary source of energy for the body; if the cells don't get sugars they will die (cells do not need protein as we are made to believe).

Complex and processed starches are hard to process and digest and require insulin to transport it to cells

Fruit sugars are simple and don't need insulin to enter the cells, they enter the cells by diffusion, fructose or fruit sugar is the highest energetic source of sugars that feed and energize cells. fruit sugars keep cells alkalized and are like little firemen putting out fires started by acids. Raw fruits and sugars are the best sources of simple sugars for your body. Complex carbs are not ideal for energy and are energy robbers-

How about vegetables
Vegetables are the builders of the body. They are great to use when you are healthy but they are not as effective for healing, this is because they are harder to digest and they don't have many astringent properties that clean the cells and the body from obstructions.

Raw veggies are the best to consume and green drinks are even better as they have no fiber and are easier to digest.
Steaming veggies is acceptable if you feel you can't consume 100% fruits when healing.

However, understand that eating cooked foods even vegetables will stop detoxification.

How To Finally Get Well Even When The World Says No

The Raw Maraby Protocol Step By Step

No matter what health issue you have you can correct the cause of the health issue by starting a detoxification program that I am about to share with you:

And yes it is a one size fits all technique. this is because 99% of all health issues will boil down to a lymphatic issue and acids- the two are tied in together and so the first step is to always change your diet from an acid ash diet (cooked foods, starches, and animal products) to an alkaline diet (raw fruits and veggies)

Also, remember that even though the body is complex in its makeup, its functioning is quite simple.

Let's put it this way- You don't need to know how a car runs to drive it. But you do know what it takes to run it. It requires fuel and oil to run it and an exhaust pipe to get rid of its waste. So long as these two parts are taken care of the car will stand the test of time.

The human cells work the same - they feed by the blood and eliminate waste by the lymphatic system.

We don't need to know how the cells work to know how to give it what it needs to work effectively.

It's very simple

Levels Of Detox You Should Be Aware Of:

When it comes to cleaning the body, repairing it and regenerating tissue, there are different levels of detoxification and they are listed in order of strength:

1.
The highest is a dry fast- this means no food and no water- this is the highest way to heal. I should point out that you should not jump to this level until you have successfully completed other levels below. It is too dangerous for some and it should be done with the right supervision and shouldn't be done alone or when one is sick.
2.
Next is water fasting- this means you can't eat food for a designated period of time you can only drink water
3.
Next is mono fruit juices- this means you pick just one fruit and you juice it. By removing the fiber you allow even easier and faster digestion- this leaves ample energy for the body to focus and heal itself. You can drink as much as you want. Just don't over drink.
4.

How to Heal Yourself Even When They Say You Can't

Mono fruit- this is the next level down- here you pick one fruit and eat nothing else but that fruit the whole day. You can have as much as you would like- Just don't overeat
5.
Fruit juices- here you can drink a mixture of juices together so long as they can be combined together, see food combining as I discussed in this book.
This is not as effective as mono fruit juices as the mixing of types of fruits creates a harder digestion period and less time for healing
6.
Fruit smoothies- these are not as effective as the rest as there are different types of fibers and fruits in one meal- it is still a powerful way to heal but not the highest.
7.
100% fruit- Here you can eat a mixture of fruits together - much like a fruit salad, just make sure that the fruits you are eating mix well with one another
9.
Fruits for breakfast and lunch and salad for dinner- also called a transition to 100% fruit. Use this for a transitioning diet if you are coming from a standard American diet or you want to take a break or slow detox when using the higher levels of detox
9.
Green drinks or smoothies
10.
Raw fruits and vegetables- a living food diet
11.
Nut, seeds, cooked veggies, leafy greens- these are not the foods or options for detox and will slow and stop detoxification- Avoid when healing at an accelerated pace.
12.
Animal products and cooked starches (grains, pasta, processed sugars)- these are not for healing and will actually reverse the healing or detoxification process- they should be avoided at all cost when healing.

Fasting

What is fasting? Fasting means the absence of water or food for a period of time. There are two kinds of fasting, dry fasting, and wet fasting. A dry fast means no food and no water. A wet fast means no food but one can drink water.

Fasting is essential because it is what nature uses to heal the body. If you keep a close look you can see animals use fasting when they are injured, a lion that gets injured will go to a corner and sleep without food or water for days to heal. Dogs do it, cats do it, and just about every living being does it.

When you are chronically ill the body will often force you into a fast. You will lose the desire to eat and drink and this is your body's way of forcing you to stop eating those foods that are hurting you. Don't wait to be forced to heal.

Why? When you fast you give the body 100% of its energy and resources to first clean, and then heal the body. There is no energy used for digestion (which requires lots of energy) and this energy is used to repair and heal the body. So when we fast we allow the body to heal itself and when combined with fruits you are doing the best you can to help the body heal itself

We use dry fasting in this protocol as it is the most effective and not as hard on the kidneys like a wet fast. Water is nature's solvent and can be acidic in an acidic body and it is hard for the kidneys especially when your body is not alkaline, the kidneys have to deal with the water you drink and so that is the reason why I don't use it in my protocol.

Use fasting to help you heal.
There are a few types of fasting:
There is a dry fast- which means no food or water for an extended period of time - usually 12 hours to 36 hours.

There is a dry fast which means no contact with water –not even washing your hands or brushing your teeth.

There is a wet-dry fast where you don't eat but take the herbal tinctures only (usually 3 times a week)

Mono fruit

Mono means one, so mono fruit means you will consume just one fruit for the entire day and nothing else. Let's say you want to have oranges today your mono fruit diet would look like this:
Breakfast: oranges
Mid breakfast: orange juice
Lunch oranges
Mid afternoon snack: oranges
Dinner: oranges

You can pick any fruit you want, but the best are citrus fruits, grapes or melons.

The mono fruit diet is great because it allows easy digestion and allows the body to heal itself

The healing crisis
When you eat fruits, the fruits will loosen mucus and help eliminate toxins and this may come out as a healing crisis. A healing crisis is a cold and flu-like symptom that occurs when the body is eliminating waste and acids. It manifests in various forms depending

on the individual. For some people, symptoms might worsen temporarily and if you are not aware of this you may take steps to suppress these symptoms thereby stopping the healing cycle.

The most common symptoms that are experienced during healing and detoxification are the following;
Skin rashes, cold and flu symptoms, gas, water retention,
irregular bowel movements, headaches, bloating, irritability, skin rashes, itching, mucus discharge, aches and pains, lack of energy(as adrenals try to recover), you may see symptoms increasing temporarily.

Moderate detox symptoms: joint pains, discharge or green and yellow mucus, urine changes color to dark brown, orange or dark yellow, chronic fatigue symptoms, racing heart, itchiness and depression

In severe cases, you might see: tumors popping out of the body, black mucus being discharged, reduced eyesight and hearing, excessive weight loss, skin splitting, loose teeth, fatigue

You have three choices when you see symptoms: become more resilient and continue using more herbs, feeding on 100% fruits and throwing in a couple of hours of dry fasting.

Or you can slow the detox down by consuming raw greens (vegetables) and salads

Or you can stop detox by eating cooked veggies.

You can also reverse or suppress detox by eating cooked starches and animal products (don't do this)

These symptoms are called "Healing crisis" for the body to detox itself it will get rid of toxins and these toxins manifest themselves with these symptoms - fruit reveals then heals. These are temporary symptoms and go away in a day or two. IEGGTf they persist consult a doctor. Cooked foods and animal products will suppress symptoms and this may give the impression that all is well when those foods are ruining your health.

Remember this "If you don't eliminate you will accumulate."
Often you can experience a worsening of symptoms, that is right every issue you might have might be expressed temporarily but it is just a temporary and you get better.

Apply caution with this and use common sense.

Proper Food Combining

How to Heal Yourself Even When They Say You Can't

There are certain foods you should not combine. This is because the body uses different enzymes to break down foods,

When you consume protein the body uses acid digestive enzymes to break these proteins down (remember that proteins are hard to digest so acids are needed to break it down).

Carbohydrates use alkaline or base enzymes to break them down.

When you eat protein and carbs you are neutralizing acids with bases and the food just sits in your stomach and ferments which then attracts fungus, parasites and bacteria

So don't combine proteins with carbs

Don't combine fruits with any other foods- ideally; don't combine fruits with even vegetables. This is because fruits digest very quickly as they are the food designed for humans and as such very little is needed to break them down. If you consume fruits with other foods, the fruit will dissolve and sit on top of the other foods and there will be fermentation and putrefaction. You get bloated and set a terrain for viruses, parasites, fungus, and bacteria.

Before we begin, we need to know what kind of fruits we can eat

Sweet fruits- dried fruit, bananas, date, figs, coconut and permissions
Acid fruits Kiwi, oranges, grapefruit, pineapple, lemon, lime, pomegranate.
Berries: black berries, blueberries, raspberries, acai.

Green drinks: Wheatgrass, spinach, dandelions, seaweed, kale, parsley. Coriander, beet tops, and bottoms.

Melons-cantaloupe, honeydew, watermelon, papaya.
 Veggie fruits-avocado, cucumber, sweet peppers, vine ripe tomatoes.

Do not eat nuts when detoxing

Avoid beans, grains, starches, and animal products
Always use organic when you can. If you can't, wash it with vinegar and baking soda.

Rules for this protocol:

- Do not eat melons with anything- they digest too fast. always eat melons and wait 45 minutes before you ingest anything else
- Do not combine protein and starches ever
- You may combine protein with vegetables

- Always go organic. Conventional fruits have too many pesticides. If you can't get organic wash your fruits with a veggie wash or a baking soda rinse. Apply 2-3 teaspoons of baking soda to a bowl of water and wash your fruits in that solution.
- Do not drink water with meals as it dilutes the digestive enzymes. You may drink water 30 minutes before or after a meal.
- Combine veggie fruits with veggies
- You may combine starches with vegetables. (don't do this when you are healing- do this on a cheat day)
- Do not combine acidic fruits with sweet fruits
- You may combine sub-acid fruits with acid fruits or sub acids acid fruits and sweet
- Always try and get your fruits to ripen. If unripe and bitter do not eat
- Drink water only when thirsty as fruits provide all the water you need
- You may eat as much fruit as you like. No calorie counting
- If you are having a salad, avoid heavy fatty dressings. Olive oil with vinegar is perfect
- Remove all cooked and processed foods
- Do not eat past 7 pm, this gives the body the needed time to digest rest and heal. If you are hungry and must eat drink juices
- By juices I don't mean pasteurized or store bought, you must drink freshly squeezed juices. You can juice and store it for 1-2 days but it has to be freshly squeezed. Store bought fruit is pasteurized and has no enzymes.
- Cheat days- This is a healing protocol so take it seriously. I know you want your health and body to be the very best possible so I do hope you have the will and strength to not cheat. However, if you do cheat on this plan, try to cheat with cooked vegetables - avoid starches and proteins. If you do cheat get right back on the plan. Don't cancel the whole day plan because you cheated on one meal
- Avoid caffeine. Drink teas that have no caffeine You must avoid coffee and any caffeine as it is acidic and will slow down your results/
  - No alcohol as well(except in tinctures)

Guidelines:

If you fall off the wagon get back on the next meal - you won't ever fail this way.
Watch proper food combination.
No calorie counting. Eat as much fruit as you want but do not overdo it. The truth is as your body detoxes you will become more efficient at digesting food and so you will not need much food. Fruits are nutrient dense and you don't need lots of it to get the nutrition you need.
Watch and expect the healing crisis.
Drink Water - drink as much as you need. Do not over drink. The fruits will hydrate you without the need for extra water, so drink only when you are thirsty. The best water is distilled water as it's free of hormones and chemicals.

The Great Lymphatic System – The Missing Key To Health And Weight Loss

Your kidneys and lymphatic system are the keys to your health. Any health issue you might be experiencing right now is due to these two. The lymphatic system is the system that removes metabolic waste from your cells and passes it on to your kidneys to get rid of. If your lymphatic system is stagnant (due to the foods you have been eating) and the kidneys are not filtering properly, health issues arise.
You may even wonder why sometimes you get fat and you can't lose the weight no matter what you do. You simply seem to be bloated and you swell (Edema) the reason for this is that your lymphatic system and kidneys are not working properly and so the body uses water to buffer the acids that are attacking cells.

If you get the kidneys and the lymphatic system to work, you will be able to get rid of waste in your body and good health is the result. Fruits are the only way to help these systems work effectively.

I want to explain this in the simplest way possible. You don't need a high school education to understand this but this is crucial for health and detox

I want you to picture a city- in the city, you have a bunch of buildings and people are living in it, these people eat every day and use the washroom, the city has a lymphatic sewer system (lymphatic system) - the main sewer system. The city takes care of this and makes sure it is working. But in each home, there are sewer pipes and toilets and these are important because if they don't move waste
into the main sewer system the waste will back up in the house and eventually kill the inhabitants of the house.
In the body the lymphatic system is the sewer system, it is in every cell or home, every home also has a kitchen as well (blood that feeds the cells). The kidneys are the main sewage management system if it breaks all the sewers and eventually, the pipes in the homes of people will break as well.

Kidney filtration

The kidneys are the sewage plant; its job is to clean the sewer.
The blood is the kitchen of the homes in the city and the septic tanks in each home or neighbourhood are the lymph nodes- these are part of the lymphatic system and their job is to clean the wastes of acids so it does not damage the kidneys. The acid level given by cells is about 3 PH the lymph nodes make it about a 6 PH, if the lymph nodes did not do this you would be peeing painfully, you would be peeling acids.

If you don't filter this out through the kidneys, the waste will back up much like a sewer system and the waste will try and come out of your skin (this is the reason why you will see skin issues, rashes, old looking skin, and hair loss), even with skin eliminating waste the lymph will back up and if left unchecked will lead to illnesses and autoimmune issues. Fruit is the only thing that can move the lymphatic system- the lymphatic system does not move like blood, it has to be stimulated to move and fruit is a way to get it moving.

How to check your urine for kidney filtration?

If you wake up in the morning pee into a clear jar, you should see sediment in the urine, it should have strings in it or cloudy like particles. If you see this you are filtering. If not you are not filtering effectively. This fruit detox program will help get your kidneys filtering

Kidney filtration tricks

You can take a small bowl with a little castor oil mix it with the cayenne powder and apply it to the skin over the top of both kidneys. You might want to rub it in really good. After that you can put on the kidneys rags that have been soaked in oil and cover it with a towel or cloth of some kind and use a heat source like a heating pad or hot water bottle

The Raw Maraby healing system (RMHS) - STEP BY STEP

Before you start an aggressive detoxification program you should always go on a transition plan like this:

Breakfast: fruits (oranges)
Lunch: fruits (grapes)
Dinner: salad with raw dressing.
Do this for 2-4 weeks.

THE RAW MARABY PROTOCOL AFTER A TRANSITION DIET

An example of a protocol

Weigh yourself and take a selfie with your camera

If you have been on a standard American diet full of meat, milk, and starches, you need to follow this pre-week program before you jump into a 100% fruit protocol. The reason for this is because your body is too constipated, too obstructed and fruit, when eaten, will dislodge all that putrid waste in your body, that waste will stir up and you will have detox effects like gas, cold and flu-like symptoms, headaches and fever these are temporary and will go away. So to minimize this we use a fruit and salad mix on the first week. You must stop all animal products and all cooked foods. No coffee, no caffeine. You will eat nothing but fruits and vegetables

Start Here:

Transition diet-Week1
Breakfast: fruits
Lunch – salad with olive oil and vinegar or any light salad dressing
Dinner- cooked vegetables simply steam any vegetables you like add spices and seasoning and enjoy.

Transition diet- Week 2
Breakfast: fruits
Lunch: fruits:
Dinner: salad

Week 1
Breakfast, lunch, and dinner – fruits
Example: You can have any combination of fruits so long as you don't mix acid fruits with sweet fruits- see food combining section
Breakfast: 5 oranges 2 tangerines
Lunch: 6 bananas and 5 dates
Dinner: 1 pound red grapes

Week 2
Breakfast, lunch, and dinner -Mono fruits
Pick one fruit and have only that fruit: it could be grapes breakfast, lunch, and dinner.

Week 3
Breakfast lunch dinner mono fruit and fruit juices
It has to be the same fruit and fruit juices for the day and no combination.

Day1
Breakfast – orange juice
Lunch -5 oranges
Dinner – orange juice
Day 2 - fruit juices all meals

Week 4-5
Day 1: fruit juices
Day 2-3: water fast
Day 4: dry fast

How to Heal Yourself Even When They Say You Can't

Day 5: fruit juices
Day 6: fruits
Repeat as you feel fit

Week 9-10
I would jump into water fasting and dry fasting if able like this:
Day 1: fruit juices
Day 2-3: water fast
Day 4: dry fast
Day 5: water fast
Day 6: dry fast
Day 7: mono fruits
Repeat as you feel fit. Continue with this protocol by repeating it as you see fit or are able to.

Remember that a dry fast means no food or water for a set period of time- a dry fast begins when sleeping as well so most people will begin their dry fast with their last meal and skip a few meals the next day. A water fast means you have no food but you can have some water as needed.

Here Is How To Detox Using Fruits

Always transition before you go 100% with fruits – remember that fruits expose weaknesses and hidden illnesses with what you are already used to a standard American diet you are full of mucus, toxins, and obstructions and detoxing too fast can throw you into a healing crisis- so use the transition plan above for a week before you start 100% fruits

There are two levels we will focus on. You have a slow detoxification program and a maximum detoxification program.
If you need to heal quickly you will want to use the maximum detox program
Here is a skeleton breakdown of how to use it for each meal

Breakfast
Use Herbal tinctures 30 minutes before meals

Freshly squeezed juice (not pasteurized) or eat one of the following:

Grapes,
mangoes,
cherries,
peaches,
pears,
bananas

Fruits
Berries (has to be organic)
Blackberries
Strawberries
Raspberries
Blueberries

Melons (Do not combine your melon with any fruit)
Watermelon
Cantaloupe
Honey dew
Papaya

Mid-morning snack

Freshly squeezed juice (not pasteurized) or eat one of the following:

Grapes,
mangoes,
cherries,
peaches,
pears,
bananas

Fruits
Berries (has to be organic)
Blackberries
Strawberries
Raspberries
Blueberries

Melons (always eat melons alone and never mix with other fruits)
Watermelon
Cantaloupe
Honey dew
Papaya

LUNCH
Use Herbal tinctures 30 minutes before meals

Mid-morning snack
Fresh fruit sugars or any one of the fruits below

Freshly squeezed juice (not pasteurized) or eat one of the following:

Grapes,
mangoes,
cherries,
peaches,
pears,
bananas

Fruits
Berries (has to be organic)
Blackberries
Strawberries
Raspberries
Blueberries

Melons (always eat melons alone and never mix with other fruits)
Watermelon
Cantaloupe
Honey dew
Papaya

Mid-afternoon snack

Freshly squeezed juice (not pasteurized) or eat one of the following:

Grapes,
Mangoes,
Cherries,
Peaches,
Pears,
Bananas

Fruits
Berries (has to be organic)
Blackberries
Strawberries
Raspberries
Blueberries

Melons (always eat melons alone and never mix with other fruits)
Watermelon
Cantaloupe
Honey dew
Papaya

Dinner
Use Herbal tinctures a 30 minutes before meals

Fresh fruit juices or any one of the fruits below

Freshly squeezed juice (not pasteurized) or eat one of the following:

Grapes,
Mangoes,
Cherries,
Peaches,
Pears,
Bananas

Fruits
Berries (has to be organic)
Blackberries
Strawberries
Raspberries
Blueberries

Melons (always eat melons alone and never mix with other fruits)
Watermelon
Cantaloupe
Honey dew
Papaya

As you can see it is very simple. You are eating fruits for breakfast, lunch, and dinner. There is nothing easier than this.

Alkalization Is The Key To Moving Lymph

When it comes to healing the body, you really need to get the body alkaline. You see the body is a predominately base (remember there are two sides to chemistry- acids and base) and. Our cells feed by the blood and excrete acidic waste via the lymphatic system, the lymph fluid is present in cells, it is in-between cells and makes about 75% of the interstitial fluid in cell- the other 25% is blood. Which makes sense as the blood feeds the cells and the lymphatic system removes the acid waste.

As the body is producing acidic waste we have to counteract by eating an alkalizing diet and alkaline foods that we have been designed for, these are the fruits.

Fruits contain minerals and sugar that alkalize a cell

When we eat acidic foods like proteins and starches, the food has to be broken down and often these foods have high amounts of protein which when broken down leaves sulphur and phosphorous which turn into sulphuric and phosphoric acid, these add to the acid burden of the cells and the entire body.

When we eat acidic ash foods the lymph fluid between cells becomes harder and it does not flow well –and this means that the acids from our 100 trillion cells have nowhere to go and begin to burn the cells, tissue, organ, and glands
True hydration does not come from fluid or water.

If you drink too much fruit juices or water, the kidneys have to regulate this water level as a result they can't focus on filtering those metabolic wastes. When you limit your fluid intake the kidneys can now focus on removing stagnant lymph. This means you should never drink when you are not thirsty. The old saying that you must drink even when you are not thirsty is untrue but also dangerous because it places a burden on the kidneys.
One of the best ways to really alkalize the cells and body is to use dried sweet fruits.

The best are figs dates and apricots. I tend to snack on dates alone as a snack in between my lemon or watermelon meals.

Dried fruits tend to have the most alkalizing nutrients that can help alkalize the body and its cells. It is compressed nutrition without the water content that gives the kidneys extra work to do.

Here is a lemon and dates protocol I often use- please note this falls in line with the raw Maraby protocol I have discussed above. Once you get the gist of proper food combination, dry fasting and herbs you can pretty much come up with your own healing protocol. And that is why goal- to show you how to heal yourself using your own combination of fruits and fasting.

Lemon And Dates Dry Fast Protocol

Last meal following day – 7 pm
Dry fast until 4 pm
Breakfast with lemon water – 1 Mason jar (32 ounces), wait 30 minutes then snack on dates (5-10 dates).

Drink lemon water again and have more dates if need, go to bed and repeat the dry fast
I could do this for 2-5 weeks straight.

Take your herbs when eating.

The Lemon Diet- Master Cleanse
I have seen this work amazingly well. This is very simple but very powerful and hard for most to follow.

You simply squeeze 2-3 lemons, a pinch of cayenne pepper and a teaspoon of agave or maple syrup mixed in 12-18 ounces of spring or distilled water and that is your meal.

You can have as much of this as you want but nothing else.

A good healing time frame is 2-4 weeks of just lemon water. Do this only if you know your capabilities and feel free to break this diet if you feel you can't do it.
You can have your herbs 30 minutes before a meal.

The Grape Diet
This is another powerful one.
You simply consume dark grapes - red or concord grapes are best and you can have as much as you want but nothing else. You will have grapes breakfast, lunch and dinner and for snacks as well.

A good healing time frame to use on the grape diet is 30-60 days.
When you eat this way you are likely to clean the body out really fast and you are not likely to get hungry after a week or two on these protocols.

You can have your herbs 30 minutes before a meal

A Powerful Dry Fasting Healing Protocol

This dry fasting/ fruits protocol is intense and heals more than anything. Do not use this if you are weak or have not done any dry fasting before.

This protocol combines dry fasting, fruits, and herbs and it is done as follows

Day 1- day 3
Eat 100% fruits and use FAB 5 tinctures three times a day
No cooked foods.
No animal products.
Its 100% fruits, good ones to use are grapes, organs, watermelon. It is best to go on mono fruit diets but you could mix them up as well.

Day 4- Dry fast- no contact with food or water

Day 5 – Break the fast you are coming out off with fresh juices and follow an hour later with 100% fruits breakfast, lunch and dinner – take FAB 5 tinctures

Day 6-day 7- 48 hours dry fast
Break the fast you are coming out off with fresh juices and follow an hour later with 100% fruits breakfast, lunch, and dinner – take FAB 5 tinctures

Day 8-day 9- 48 hour feed with 100% fruits

How to Heal Yourself Even When They Say You Can't

Day 10-day 13- 72 hours dry fast. Break the fast you are coming out off with fresh juices and follow an hour later with 100% fruits breakfast, lunch, and dinner – take FAB 5 tinctures.

Day 14-day 17 100% fruits. Break the fast you are coming out off with fresh juices and follow an hour later with 100% fruits breakfast, lunch and dinner – take FAB 5 tinctures

DAY 18-DAY20 Dry fast.

Day 21-day 24 100% fruits break the fast you are coming out off with fresh juices and follow an hour later with 100% fruits breakfast, lunch, and dinner – take FAB 5 tinctures

Day 29-30 Dry fast.

Break the fast you are coming out off with fresh juices and follow an hour later with 100% fruits breakfast, lunch, and dinner – take FAB 5 tinctures

You can go as long as you can go to heal yourself. Some healing can take 6 months to 2 years so just learn how to use this super powerful healing protocol and play with it

A Water Fast Protocol

Water fasting is very intense but you will get the desired result which is total healing. But should be done only after a month of 100% fruits to clean out the body before an intense fast,

Water fast means you have no solid food but should include herbs and herbal tea (no caffeine). Use distilled or spring water only.

Start with 24 hour water fast, and then build up all the same to 21-30 day water fast
Don't do this protocol if you are not strong enough or are too weak or have never fasted before as it can be dangerous

The herbs are a huge part of the water fast; the herbs will help clean out cells intestinally and remove obstructions to health- uses the FAB5 tinctures as discussed below.

The Orange Mucus Buster Protocol

This protocol is simple, you need to stick to lemons, oranges, and grapefruit and herbs- use the Fab 5 tinctures, use the GI cleanser (recipe found in later chapter below) for a few weeks,
You make the mucus buster orange juice like this:

Squeeze 4-5 oranges, plus grapefruit+ 1 to 2 lemons+ add a few drops of stevia if need

Drink this as often as you like. You can't have any cooked food with this protocol; it is 100% raw fruits as I have spelled out below
It is a diet of oranges, lemon, and grapefruit
It looks like this:

Fab 5 herbs (herbs for the adrenals, kidneys, lymph, bowels, and endocrine) at 11 am

Breakfast after 12 pm
Orange juice only

Snack 3-4 oranges

Fab 5 herbs (herbs for the adrenals, kidneys, lymph, bowels, and endocrine) at 11 am

Lunch 4 oranges

Snack mucus buster drink

Fab 5 herbs (herbs for the adrenals, kidneys, lymph, bowels, and endocrine) at 11 am

Dinner: oranges.

As you can see all the protocols all fall in line with the raw Maraby protocol guidelines

The 45-60 day grape fast

This one is my favorite with desperate cases; for people who really want to heal. I call it – the desperate healing protocol. To use this you need to use a transition diet (see transition diet above) for at least a week, before you jump into a 40 day/40-night grape diet.

The daily eating schedule will look like this:
Do a dry fast from your last meal for 14 hours
Then
Breakfast: grapes – eat as much as you want
Snack: grape juice or grapes
Lunch: grapes
Snack: grape juice or grapes
Dinner: grapes

Prepare a GI cleaner cleanse drink and drink it daily.
Use the FAB 5 tinctures 3 times a day 30 minutes before a meal. Don't use tinctures during a dry fast as you are fasting.
Do a daily enema after the dry fast

How to Heal Yourself Even When They Say You Can't

Every 5 days do a 24 hour dry fast- where you eat no food or drink no water. Break that fast with grapes.

Although I have said 45-60 days grape fast, you can go on this protocol as long as you would like or until you feel well.

Tools You Need For Healing

The GI Tract Is Another Key To Detoxification

The GI tract makes up the entire passageway from your head to your anus and it connects all the important organs together. It also comprises the bowel and the small and large intestine, these all need to be cleaned out.

If you don't clean the GI tracts when you are cleaning the lymphatic system, the waste can be returned back into the bloodstream so it's crucial that they are cleaned,

A 100% fruit diet will clean it out but we can also use a GI cleaner as explained below which helps scrape the walls of the GI tract

Once you have cleaned the bowels you will be able to absorb the nutrients you digest. It just makes sense to clean the bowels and GI tract.

GI Tract Cleaner

Put the following ingredients into a glass

- 1 tbsp. Bentonite Clay (makes sure it is aluminum and lead-free)
- 1 tbsp. Whole or powdered Psyllium Husk
- 1 teaspoon activated charcoal
- 12 ounces of water

Add some cold water or juice to the mixture and stir to make a paste. Gulp it down quickly before it turns into oatmeal like consistency. Drink another glass of water. After ingesting this "cleaner."

Drink this daily at first and then build up to 2-3 times a day. If you are constipated do not use this cleanser until you are somewhat regular.

Enemas and colonics

Enemas are important when it comes to healing. This is because you want to remove any fecal matter that is sitting dormant in the colon. A colonic done by a professional once a month is also helpful. Remember that the bowels and the entire GI tract are crucial when it comes to health as every organ is connected to it and so you want to get toxins out of the bowels.

You can find an enema bag with instructions from any health food store. Do not put chemicals in the enema bag (some health stores give you free solutions to put into the enema bag and you don't want this).
Use distilled or spring water in your enema bag, you can put a shot of freshly squeezed wheatgrass otherwise just use distilled water.

The GI cleanser is also very important because we do fasting and a fruit protocol, the acids, sulphur, plaque, parasites all get dislodged and so taking a GI cleanser will help remove those loose unwanted material out of the body so it doesn't reabsorb in the bloodstream.

Are you worth it?

What if you knew that you could follow a simple protocol and get better would you not do it?

If I told you to invest $75 on a bottle of herbs and commit for 2-3 weeks and just maybe, maybe you will see great strides in your health would you not give it a try?

I hope YES is your answer because good health is priceless.

Well, my friends, I have done that for you- the key to health is right here in this book and you have now read it and all you need to do is implement it.

I have literally given you the key to health...I have often wondered why people who have discovered great things like Tesla with free electricity. Tesla in his knowledge had the knowledge for free electricity and yet was not able to give everyone unlimited electricity. The secret died with him and one might ask, "Why did he not share it with every man and woman on earth?"

I am sharing my knowledge with you right here. **I am doing it right here, this health** system I am sharing is so simple and yet so effective your mind might say healing cannot be this simple.

However, it is up to you- ignore the doubt and try this and see for yourself. You be the proof and then decide.

The great treasures of life are simple, they are also in plain sight, and in fact, sometimes so obvious yet we miss them because of our ego and over intellectualism. This healing protocol with fruits is the same thing- so simple, many intellectuals will miss it. They will argue about this theory and that theory. I really don't care, what I do care is that you heal and if this book puts you in the right direction I have done my part

Here is the formula again:

How to Heal Yourself Even When They Say You Can't

Fruits + herbs + patience (action) is the key to abundant health- if you choose to follow it you will benefit, if you ignore it you have **only you** to blame in the end.

Life After Detox- How To Eat After Detox

So how long do you go on fruits? How long do you keep doing this?

There is such a thing as a fruitarian lifestyle where you eat nothing but fruits. Fruits supply all the nutrients amino acids and carbohydrates you need so you could be a fruitarian or a vegan like me where I eat 90% fruits and 10% vegetables. Sometimes I will also have cooked vegan meals as well. It is all about balance. If you still wish to eat meat after this I don't recommend it as it's the cause of the health issues, to begin with. However, it is your choice and as you know how to heal you can decide when you need to detox or not.

In your own time, you will find out the best lifestyle that promotes good health is a raw vegan diet and not processed or animal products.

Mental strength and will power - This Is Important
Find your why.
Keep away from negative social circles

How to succeed at detox

Some of us are in this journey by choice others are here by necessity. In both cases, it's essential to learn how to get the drive so you don't quit.

Step 1:
Find your why and know your goal - write it down in detail.

Step 2:
Go all in and decide to do this.

Step 1: get emotional. When you put emotion behind your goals and your why you tend to succeed.

Step 3: small steps on a daily basis creates momentum

Step 4: results - evaluate each day - did you move forward - if not why not?

Your why will make you emotional if not find the right one - it's your fuel if you don't have it you will fail.

Don't let failures or cheats on your diet take you off track, always jump right back onto fruits the next meal- Remember that it's a journey, not a destination.

FAQ ABOUT A FRUIT DIET:

Question: How do I start?

Simply replace what you would ordinarily eat at breakfast, lunch and/or dinner with fruits.

Breakfast: Orange juice and oranges
Lunch: Melon
Dinner: Grapes, or if you crave greens, raw vegetables and raw salad with a raw salad dressing.
You can mix and match your fruits; just don't mix sweet fruits with acidic fruits, and don't mix melons with any other fruit. As these fruits are digested at different rates.

Question: How much should I eat a day?
There is no calorie counting when eating a 100% fruit diet. I like to avoid avocados and coconuts, as they are heavy and not the best detoxifiers. But, by all means, have them if you are hungry.

Question: I get hungry all day; what should I eat?

Eat fruit when you are hungry. Having seven or eight oranges with you is a good idea, as when you are hungry you can peel and eat one.

Question: Should you squeeze your own juice or buy it in stores?

Always squeeze your own juice. Store-bought juice is pasteurized, and this means every enzyme has been destroyed. Some stores do offer freshly squeezed juices and you can use that—just make sure it is fresh and squeezed the same day. Juice is really only good for a few hours; after that time, it loses much of its nutrition and energy or life force.

Question: Can I use nonorganic fruits?

Yes, you can. Just wash your fruit with a baking soda wash. You simply add one teaspoon of baking soda to a bowl of water, put your uncut fruits in it and let them soak for 15 minutes. Then, rinse off the fruit, place it in the fridge and eat it, as needed.

Question: I feel intimidated and I don't know where to start—what should I do first?

This is simple: To get yourself started, just try a three-day grape-only diet. For three days, eat only grapes and nothing else. You can have grapes for breakfast, lunch and dinner. Once you complete three days, you can try to add more "grape only" days to it. You can eat and consume as many grapes as you want. You will realize that this will build your confidence and show you the power of fruits in healing. This will encourage you to get into a fruit diet for a longer period of time.

Question: How do I shop for fruits…or what fruits should I buy?

Any fruit will do—buy fruits you have available to you; if you can't find any fresh fruits, use frozen organic fruits and make a smoothie. It is that simple to start a fruit diet!

Question: Should I juice or eat my fruit?

Juicing is more effective, as there is less digestion and therefore less energy is used by the body in digestion, so more energy and enzymes are left for healing. You can juice and eat fruits on the same day.

Question: What times should I have my fruits?

Anytime! Eat when you're hungry, and if you are eating 100% fruits, you can eat as much as you want—there is no calorie counting.

Question: How much fruit can I eat?

There is no calorie counting when on a 100% fruit diet, although "less is more," as less means that your body has less to digest. Eat until you are satisfied and eat whenever you are hungry.

Question: How long should I go on a fruit diet or detox program?

You can go on a fruit diet or detox program for as long as needed. The time frame varies for each person, but in general, a 14-week protocol is a great detox period for most. You might detox for more time if you are healing a tough condition.

Question: Is fruit acidic? If so, can I eat acidic fruits?

Acidic fruits like citrus fruits are the most healing and, when consumed, leave an alkaline hit to the body. Just because a fruit is an acidic fruit does not mean it is bad for you. Meat, for instance, is neutral in pH when uncooked, but when ingested, it is highly acidic to the body.

Question: What fruits can I have? Can I have a fruit bowl and what can I combine?

Here are the rules of fruit combinations:

The sweet fruit category includes the following: banana, date, fig, sapote, persimmon, cherimoya, carob, Mammea fruit, plantain, sapodilla, sugar apple, etc.
All of these fruits can be paired with all other fruits, with the exception of acidic fruits and melons.

Acidic fruits include the following: Blackberry, orange, passion fruit, strawberry, tangerine, tomato (technically a fruit), ugli fruit, grapefruit, acerola cherry, and Pineapple.

The "sub acid" fruit category includes fruits like the following: Apple, papaya, peach, pear, raspberry, ugli fruit, apricot, blackberry, blueberry, grape, cherry, mango, mulberry, nectarine, tamarillo, and guava. Sub acid fruits pair well with all non-sweet fruits.

It is no surprise that melons have a category to themselves—eat melons alone, "without mixing them with other fruits.
The fat category of fruits includes the following: avocado, durian, coconut, and akee.

Can Kids use this?
Yes, fruits are essential for kids. There is no sense in pumping your kids with processed foods, cooked starches, and animal protein. It is too acidic for them and often leads to illnesses, weight gain, allergies, and immune issues.

All this can be avoided by eating raw fruits and veggies. Now I know some kids will be very difficult and won't allow such a change but you can gradually introduce raw fruits and veggies and help them get used to fruits and veggies,

Kids naturally and instinctively love fruits, some kids already have congested lymph thanks to their parents' diet before, during and after birth. So kids will take on a burdened lymph system, poor kidneys and a taste of chemicals and additives, but this is all reversible.

Feed your kids fruit meals when you can.
A good diet schedule on fruits for a child would be for most days (not being extreme)

Day 1
Breakfast: Orange juice)
Lunch (Oranges)
Dinner: avocado and salad

Day 2
Same

Day 3
Fruit juices only

Repeat

Once a week they will fast 12 hours build up to 24 hours
Insert "cheat" (social events or traditional dinners) days randomly.

Time is needed for healing
A lot of people will eat all the wrong foods for years, they will abuse their bodies and when they finally get unwell they expect to get well and to heal the body in a few days. This is not realistic. The body is a very powerful and resilient machine, meaning that it can take decades of abuse but when it has had enough it is going to tell you through sicknesses.

To remove the obstructions in the body it can take time- for serious cases, 6 months to a year is a good number.

For acute or sub-acute cases a 2-4 months plan will do wonders.

You will, however, always see improvements in a few days and weeks of getting on fruits dry fasting and herbs. Think of this as a journey and not a goal and you will feel your life, sprit and health transform with fruits and herbs.

Is the raw fruit protocol realistic?
Yes, it is the absolute best way to heal the body. This is what the human body was designed to eat as we are a tropical species. Once you get into this you will feel better and look amazing.

QUESTION: Is this practical long term?

Yes, first heal yourself with 100% fruits and once you are healed you can go back to some cooked vegan or veggies as well.
And remember when things get bad, health wise in the future, one looks back and says "I wish I had done this or listened "

Nothing is drastic unless you say so and either way it's your duty to show kids the better choice and avoid following the crowd to make the wrong decisions. Yes maybe it may be severe but you can implement 70% of it and in time common sense and results will tell you what you are doing is right. This applies to everything - nothing is hard we are just too comfortable in our comfort zone.

How can this fruit protocol be a one size fits all?

Yes, this is so because generally, the body gets sick due to obstructions. And no matter the symptom, it is a cause and effect situation. You have caused this obstruction and the symptoms are expressed in places that are genetically weak.

For a body to be well, it has to have proper digestion, absorption, utilization, and elimination. If any of these are obstructed there will be a problem.

Literally, you are sick because you are full of waste.. To get all obstruction out eat a fruit diet (mono fruit), use herbs or botanicals and add some dry fasting (24-36 hours) in between the fruits. Just try it and see. The proof is in the pudding. However, you can't go from meat direct to only fruit- there has to be a few days transition as fruit dislodges toxins and if you are clogged up inside it can be an issue as these wastes tend to leech back into the blood and vital systems of the body.

Sugar and Candida

There is a misconception that fruits feed fungi, and bacteria and this is not true.
You have to understand the purpose of fungus and bacteria in nature. They are mature janitors or garbage men, their job are to come and the breakdown and break up foods that we can't digest. Some bacteria are called protein splitters, meaning they will come and split up protein that can't be digested. When we eat cooked foods like proteins and starches, the body can't break down these "foods" effectively, so this means those foods rot in the body and ferment, and invites bacteria and fungus.
Fermentation and rotten foods create the opportunity of these bacteria and fungi to breed

When we eat fruits, we are eating very simple and easy to digest food and this food doesn't sit and ferment because it takes about 20-40 minutes to breakdown these foods, compare that to protein and complex carbohydrates which can take up to 8 hours to digest, leaving lots of opportunity for the food to ferment and encourage these fungi and bacteria

Remember that the fungal and bacteria family is a "fermented sugar" family. They will grow in or on fermented foods like bread, cheeses and undigested protein, Fungus will only grow on fruit when it's overly ripe and breaking down- fungus won't attack ripe fruit.

Getting 100% fruits and adding herbs is an effective way of dealing with Candia, yeast issues and bacterial overgrowths.

These creatures come when there is fermentation and won't affect the body if the body is kept clean and there are no undigested foods for it to break down and clean out

Sugar and cancer

There is a myth out there that sugars feed cancer and this is not true. Understand what a cancer cell is, it is a damaged cell. It is a cell that is breaking down and that has been trapped in an acidic medium with nowhere to go (the body can't remove it as the body or area has become too hard, dry and blocked the flow of energy that it normally uses it to clean dead cells)

An acidic body and ketosis will damage cells and a damaged cell is on its way to becoming A-typical cell to say that sugar feeds cancer is to say that vegetables, animal products, and complex carbohydrates also contain sugars and therefore will feed cancer as well. Fructose is a simple sugar and is very nurturing and anti-inflammatory to a cell. They are also alkalizing and remember acidosis or acidity is what causes cancer and you need alkalizing nutrients and sugars from fruit sugars to put out the inflammation or fires in the body that acidosis creates.
Fruits will also get your lymphatic system moving and clean which is the system that deals with removing acids and dead cells from the body as well.

Fruits are high antioxidants as well

Fructose does not require insulin to make its way to cells and fruits also don't require extensive digestive enzymes to be used, which allows the body the resources and time it needs to heal. Fruits have magnetic energy which makes them nerve foods and will bring energy to the body - most foods like animal protein and cooked starches tend to rob the body of energy. So never fear the use of fruits to heal

Will fruits give me diabetes?

No. Fruit sugar enters a cell by diffusion which means there is not much need for insulin. Protein, carbohydrates, and starches need insulin and are also acidic. These create an acidic environment which causes inflammation which affects the pancreas and the adrenal glands.
Fruits will help rebuild the pancreas and adrenal glands which are the glands that are the main causes of diabetes and obesity

Too much sugar in fruits?

This is not true; there is more sugar in 100 grams of white bread than 100 grams of sweet banana. Sure they taste sweet but they have less sugar than complex carbohydrates

Refined processed sugar is dangerous and addictive but should not be compared with fructose or fruit sugars,

Starchy foods like pasta, rice, yams, bread, and flour are also sugars and they tend to be very hard to digest for the body and they need lots of insulin to be used by the cells for energy.

Fruits contain a sugar called fructose, Fruits are easy to digest and essential in healing the cells, tissue and the body as a whole

Remember that your body is a complex machine and like all machines, it needs fuel or energy to run. And to function, we need to give the body amino acids, fatty acids, and sugars.
However, it should be known that sugar mixed with oxygen is what fuels the body

Let's discuss the two types of sugars- these are monosaccharide and polysaccharides:

Monosaccharide is known as simple sugars, examples are glucose (sugars from vegetables), fructose (from fruit sugar), or galactose (this comes from milk sugar). It should be known that a simple sugar cannot be broken down any further to be used.

Poly or Disaccharides are known as complex sugars- you will find these in starches and complex carbohydrates. These sugars contain several glucose/fructose bonds. They are therefore very hard to digest when compared to fruit sugars.

This is crucial in seeing why fruit sugars are a better choice for sugars than complex sugars. complex carbohydrates must be broken into simple sugars before the body can use them- this can take hours to digest and it demands high energy and resources form the body to use- this means the body is being robbed of the energy to break down food for energy- it simply makes no sense.

So when you consume starches the body has to deal with an overload of simple sugars that it has broken down, this leaves excess sugars in the bloodstream and there is now a high demand on the pancreas to produce insulin and a high demand on the liver and kidneys to use and or eliminate any excess.

If the body can't deal with these excess sugars it can create serious health issues.

There are no proteins in fruits and veggies

This is false. As a society, we are brainwashed into thinking that we need protein from animal products but this is not true. All the most powerful creatures on earth eat vegetables and fruits and they don't seem to need "animal products". A buffalo, an elephant, apes, and gorillas don't eat meat. Their diet is made of greens and fruits. The only animals that eat animal proteins are carnivores and we don't look or digest like them. Think about it- if all animals needed complex protein likes animal protein we would not have any animals in existence except carnivores

Protein is a complex structure that is very difficult for the body to break. When you consume animal protein you are eating dead and rotten flesh that offers no bio-available nutrients. Bio-available means the body can readily use the protein without the need of complex chemistry to tear down or break the protein, animal protein offers no bio-available protein, the body has to break down the protein to the amino acids it needs but in so doing it leaves an acid ash deposit.

FAQ
QU: Fruits have too Much Sugar.

Fruit sugars are not like refined sugars. They are not inflammatory and they don't hurt the body. The sugars in fruit don't need much insulin to get into a cell compare this with proteins and complex carbohydrates which need insulin. This alone should tell you how much better fruits are as an energy source than animal proteins and complex carbohydrates. Fruits are high nutrition foods. They are filled with antioxidants, minerals, and vitamins. Some are astringent and help dissolve and liquefy hard mucus. Fruits are nurturing and healing and highly alkaline and among all foods, they offer the most energy to cells.

And do not be fooled, you can consume a plate of pasta and it has more sugar than a plate of fruit. Not all sugars are the same. Fruit sugars are good and healing to the body.

Fruit sugars are not a cause of diabetes, inflammation is. when we eat foods that are acidic and foreign to the human body such as protein and starches the body becomes acidic or inflamed and the result is an immune response by the body - this immune response or acidity if left uncared for will eventually lead to inflammation and this can affect glands such as the pancreas which is the gland that produces insulin causing diabetes.

Inflammation is from acidosis and acidosis is from eating alien food to the food which is animal proteins, cooked foods, cooked starches, and processed foods. Fruits if given the chance can nurture the glands to good health.

Of course, always see your doctor if you are embarking on a diet change or new health program as only they will know if you are able to get on more fruits and vegetables

QU: Can I gain weight/ build muscle on this?

If your goal is to gain weight and muscle mass. You should first clean yourself out with this health protocol; you need to remove mucoid plaque and obstructions that are causing mal-absorption. Once you are clean you can go on high-calorie fruits such as: Avocados, coconut flesh, figs and dates to bulk up.

Remember to build a new house you need to fix the foundation and so going on a detoxification program before you bulk up with fruits is a good idea. So use the protocol in this book, clean your body and then bulk up.

I will get too skinny on fruits

When you go on a detox sometimes you may lose weight and for some people who are already thin, they get concerned.

This is an issue that needs to be discussed.

When you detox, you are tearing down all of which the body has stored and does not need. What will happen often is that the body because it can't get rid of waste effectively will store the toxins in body fat.

It will also hold water weight to buffer acids
Remember that there are 4 paths ways the body will eliminate waste
1. The colon
2. The kidneys
3. The skin
4. The lungs

If any of these pathways of elimination are obstructed the body is going to hold weight. So when you get on a detox program and actually get the body working again, you are going to lose excess or toxic waste.

Add to that there is the issue of mal-absorption.

Mal-absorption means you are not absorbing nutrients- the small intestines have tiny hair-like structures that pick up nutrients from digested food when you are obstructed with mucoid plaque on the bowel walls, this hair like structures can't absorb food as they are sealed and blocked by undigested proteins and starches. This prevents you from getting enough nutrients and from gaining weight. You will find yourself eating lots of food but not being able to gain weight.

However, when you detox and remove this mucoid plaque you will be able to gain or lose weight far easier and healthier than ever before because you would have removed that obstruction to energy flow and health.

Here is the weird part, the very same diet you are on that will have you lose weight will be the very same diet that will put muscle and weight back on when you are done healing- showing you that it is not the calories or type of food, but it is the body eliminating waste and then healing itself.

So don't worry about looking too thin, it will pass as the body fixes itself. Remember, to build a skyscraper you need to tear down the existing structure and put a proper foundation. Then and only then can you build.

Motivation

Never give up, stay consistent. If you cheat on this protocol don't get derailed - get back on the tracks. Think of it this way

You've already committed and won half the battle by getting on the train. So as long as you stay on the train you will make it to your destination. One easy step leads to many miles. Before you begin your journey seems long into it, you realize you are already half way through.

The Tongue Test

You can tell if you have acids –eyes, ears, clogged, sinus issues. Do the tongue test to use the tongue method, dry fast for one day or eat fruits for 2-3 days and nothing else, if your tongue coats with a heavy residue it reflects how much stagnation and obstruction you have. It is an indication of the toxins and impurities in the body.

So You Have A Health Problem What Do You Do?
First, always see a doctor if it is an emergency. This is about healing and not treating. My goal is to educate yourself so you can heal yourself but always use good judgment and common sense and see a doctor before you embark on any health protocol

There are thousands of symptoms and health issues but they are all viewed the same in detoxification. Don't take my word for it, simply hydrate the body and remove the acids that cause dehydration and you will see that I am speaking the truth.

You see the cause of the issue is acids that block energy flow. Once you know the cause of these acids (cooked starched and animal products) and you replace these foods with hydrating foods that the human species was designed to eat (fruits) and watch how your health transforms.

The proof is in you, for if you use this simple method of healing you will see your health improving and health issues go away.

Some chronic health issues will take 6-24 months to clean up but it can be done.

Summary

What it takes to heal and detoxify the body.

Step 1

How to Heal Yourself Even When They Say You Can't

Change your diet from an acid ash diet to an alkaline diet (100% raw fruits and veggies)

Step 2

Fix the 4 processes of digestion, absorption, utilization, and elimination by using 100% fruits and herbs. Use herbs for the adrenals. Kidneys, lymph, endocrine and stomach, and bowels- we call this the Fabulous 5 or Fab 5.

No matter what the health issue and if you are trying to heal with fruits and herbs, you always, always go on the Fab 5 tinctures. There is no one out there who does not have weak adrenals, kidneys, lymph system, endocrine and stomach, and bowels. So you will benefit by taking these herbs whilst on a raw food diet.

It is the foundation of the 4 processes of getting well I explained above, which are digestion, absorption, utilization, and elimination.

Think of herbs as an investment and not a cost. Most people will waste money on junk food, movies and other things that bring no benefit and yet complain that they can't afford fruits and herbs. And in the Fab 5. I have given you every single herb needed for those systems to operate better in conjunction with a 100% raw fruit diet.

Step 3

Stick to it- a good way to heal fast is to get on a 20-30 grape or lemon diet as this follows the 100% raw fruits requirement

Step 4

Stick to it- remember that your health issues did not just appear, it took years to manifest and detoxification as powerful as it is, it will require time to allow the body to heal itself. Time is needed, a good detox time frame for acute and sub-acute issues are 12-14 weeks and 6 months to 2 years for chronic and degenerative cases. But in all cases, you are going to see improvements in days of using this protocol.

Examples. These are for educational purposes only.

John can't lose weight, he has tried everything and being to his doctor and the doctor has said there is nothing to be done, it is his thyroid.

What should John do?

John should switch his diets to 100% fruits

How to Heal Yourself Even When They Say You Can't

John should use herbs that address the 4 processes - digestion, absorption, utilization and elimination- He should use the FAB 5 herbs.

Just because his thyroid is not functioning properly does not mean the thyroid is the problem.

The problem is acids and we know that when acids can't be eliminated the backup and burn cells and glands (thyroid) so if we can get those acids out we can get better

So John has to get his lymph moving with fruits and get the kidneys filtering with dry fasting and herbs.

If he does this the acids will leave and the thyroid can heal itself.

See how simple it is?

Example2.

Jane has high blood pressure. She is taking medication from her doctor but Jane wants to stop them and told her doctor that she is changing her diet.

We know that acids are responsible, for acids affect the kidney and adrenals and these control blood pressure. And we know why these acids are damaging these glands because they are stuck, so we take steps to remove those acids by fixing our lymphatic system and kidneys so the acids can leave.

Here is what Jane did:

She went on a 30-day fruit diet. She stopped eating any cooked foods

She took herbs for the 4 processes- The Fab 5.

She did some dry fasting

Jane is healing and her doctor has taken her off her medication.

Balding protocol

Baldness and hair loss is a sign of disease. It is a sign of acidosis. It is a very serious issue as these same acids causing the hair loss is also affecting the brain and can and will set you up for Dementia, Parkinson, and Alzheimer's.

Dandruff is the same, those flakes as dried lymph fluid forcing its way out of the scalp- it is proof that your kidneys are not working properly, it is an indication that adrenals are down and most likely the GI tract is also compromised.

Think of Chemotherapy and you will understand what balding is, it is as a result of acids burning hair follicles, chemo burn's hair follicles and acids from your cells will also burn hair follicles.

So you need to get the body alkaline and get those acids out, otherwise, they will harden lymph and stop the lymphatic system from removing acids that burn tissue, organ, and glands.

You need to give 6-12 months for this to really work. You need to use the Fab 5 herbs and upper circulation for 6-12 months- hair does take time to grow but it also takes time to clean out the GI tract and body especially from a bald head- the great part of this is that you will be improving your healthy skin and hair will grow as you get healthier

When I say balding is not genetic I mean to say that you are not doomed if your family has balding in their history. It is more accurate to say you have a genetic lymphatic issue in the scalp region, however it is also true that you can grow it back with the right detoxification program. You simply need to stick to a 100% fruits diet coupled with the use of the FAB tinctures and the upper circulation tinctures.

- Do dry fast sessions to get the kidneys filtering
- Hydrate with fruits (when not fasting)
- Use upper circulation herbs. (See resource section).
- Use brain and nerves 2 herbs (See resource section).
- Use the Fab 5 tinctures.
- Get rid of sinus congestion with ear candling
- Fix kidneys, adrenals, and lymph by using tonics and herbs.
- Use hot and cold compressions. If hair does not re-grow then it means there is a problem and you need to dig deeper with the detox. Hair will grow once you are free of obstructions.

You will often notice that those who are balding initially will have sinus issues, sometimes nasal polyps, phlegm, nose, and ears issues- these are signs that the body is trying to remove this congestion and obstruction due to lymph stagnation. Mucus is tied to the mucosa which is tied to the lymph system

- Clear the mucous from the head –the sinus to clear sinuses you have to clean your head which sits on the GI tract and kidneys need to the filer
- Clean bowels-get cellular hydration (fruits and fruit juices), mucus will come out and hair will grow.
- Stop consuming acid ash forming foods. This means stop eating cooked foods starches. Protein and all animal products or animal-based foods... replace these meals with fruits only.

Skin issues- how to get rid of them through detox.

In natural healing, the skin is called the third kidney and it is the largest organ of the body. The body will try and pass acids through the skin when the two kidneys aren't functioning properly. So it is a good idea to get the skin healthy as well as detoxify the kidney and the entire body for that matter.

Skin issues like psoriasis and eczema are lymphatic and kidney issues, the body can't get rid of metabolic waste through the lymphatic system and through to the kidneys so it uses the skin which then expresses those acids as damage to the skin. In natural healing, you can't treat these conditions as they are internal conditions

The redness you see on your skin is acids trying to burst out.

Solution:

Go on 100% fruits- a 30-40 day grape fast with some dry fasting will do wonders or just follow the protocol above step by step and use the Fab 5 tinctures as well.

Clean the GI tract, the GI tract connects every organ from the head to the anus and it is crucial that it is not blocked or full of mucoid plaque. You can clean the GI tract by using the Fab 5 herbs on a 100% raw fruit diet. You can also use a GI tract cleaner as I shared with you above.

For wrinkles- this is a parathyroid issue as the parathyroid is responsible for skin elasticity and tissue strength, it is what makes use of calcium and when it is not functioning properly you will see wrinkles and other calcium deficiencies occur- a parathyroid glandular and the protocol above will go a long way in improving the skin and wrinkle appearance.

Take Advantage Of Botanicals

Remember at the start of my book I said that health issues are caused by the disruption of the mucous membrane and obstruction of energy flow? And that the first step is to clean the cells of the body and the second step is to re-energize the body. Well, we re-energize the body with alkaline fruits but we also energize with herbs. Herbs are non-hybrid foods that contain electrical and magnetic energy. Their purpose is to help strengthen, clean and re-energize the cells.

And they do it so well.

Herbs are a gift from nature, in fact, you will see that some plants resemble specific body parts, organs, and glands and that those herbs help those tissues heal. Herbs are the real medicine and they have been used since the beginning of time and science is only now catching up to it. If you go to PubMed and put the name of any of the thousands of herbs in there you will find actual scientific studies behind them so don't believe for one moment that herbs are some made up science since they are the real deal. Most pharmaceutical drugs are modeled from plants- they are the chemical version of the plant. Aspirin, for instance, was modeled after the white willow bark. White willow is safe, natural and good for you.

Herbs are tissue-specific; this means there are herbs for the kidneys, lymph system, the liver, and the endocrine systems

When detoxing, it is a great idea to use for the adrenals.kidneys, lymph system, endocrine and stomach and bowels (GI tract). I call it the Fab 5.

Use this no matter what your goal is when it comes to detoxification. This is because these organs and glands are crucial in the 4 processes of getting well- which I explained above - Digestion, absorption, utilization, and elimination. If you don't fix these processes you will have a hard time healing. These herbs also re-energize or recharge cells and allow you to get healthy rather quickly.

So always use the Fab 5 tinctures to heal. It is not an expense, it is an investment. Think for a second, you probably buy stuff you don't need, you spend money on vices that are harming you, so making a sacrifice and investing in herbs is a must if you really want to heal. Here are the herbs you need for the Fab 5:

ADRENAL GLAND

Chaste Tree Berry
Cleavers Herb
Dandelion Root & Leaf
Eleuthero Root
Ho Shou Wu Root
Holy Basil
Juniper Berry
Kelp
Parsley (whole)
Rhodiola Root
Saw Palmetto Berry
Wild Yam Root
Wild Yam Root

BOWELS

Cape Aloe Leaf
Cascara Sagrada Bark 15% by Volume
Fennel Seed
Gentian Root
Ginger Root
Plantain Leaf
Slippery Elm Bark
White Oak Bark
Wild Yam Root

ENDOCRINE

Astragalus Root
Bee Propolis Powder
Chaste Tree Berry
Eleuthero Root
Ho Shou Wu Root
Kelp Fronds Powder
Parsley (whole)
Prickly Ash Bark
Saw Palmetto Berry
Suma Root
Wild Yam Root

KIDNEY

Cordyceps
Corn Silk
Couch Grass Root
Dandelion Leaf
Goldenrod
Horsetail Herb
Juniper Berry
Parsley Leaf
Stinging Nettle Leaf

LYMPH

Chaparral Herb -replace with Blue Violet Leaf or Blue Flag
Cleavers Herb

Echinacea Root
Plantain Leaf
Poke Root
Prickly Ash Bark
Red Root
White Oak Bark

To Summarize:

I wrote this book to help you heal. I wrote it so you have no excuses whatsoever. A lot of people complain about different health issues, but the truth is that it doesn't really matter what kind of sickness it is because it all boils down to inflammation and obstructions to energy flow. In all those cases, addressing the four processes (digestion, absorption, utilization, and elimination) discussed earlier will help remove the root cause of the problem. ,,

So to heal in summary here is what you do:

1. Change your diet and go on 100% raw fruits and herbs and use tissue-specific herbs to heal. Pick a detoxification level that is good for you. E.g. dry fasting, juice diet, etc.

2, Stick to it and enjoy. You need to give your body time to heal. While, you will see immediate improvements for tough issues a good amount of time is needed, 6-24 months.

So remember this is healing and not treatment, if your condition is bad, you should go see a doctor, there is no reason why you can't see a doctor whilst taking responsibility for your health and healing yourself naturally after he or she has treated you.

I hope you enjoyed this book, I want you to apply the principles you have learned from this book because it wouldn't make any sense if you just read and don't practice it. Help heal yourself so you can help those around you with fruits and herbs. And if this book helped you please do share with another person who you care about think may need help.

Resources

Get the herbs here https://miraherbals.info/collections/product-for-health

Reach me on social media and feel free to ask questions:
On Join us on Facebook to learn how to heal: https://facebook.com/miraherbals
Ask questions on healing here https://www.instagram.com/raw_maraby/
YouTube: Search for Raw maraby
Tik tok http://vm.tiktok.com/acgaXK/
Pinterest: https://pinterest.ca/miraherbalsinc

Where to reach us: shop for the best skin and hair care products on the market here
https://miraherbals.info

How to Heal Yourself Even When They Say You Can't

Made in United States
North Haven, CT
29 April 2024